Nature's Solution for Healthy Hair

7 Ayurvedic Herbs for 100% Hair Regrowth Anyone Can Use to Overcome Baldness, Alopecia, Thinning and Other Conditions

Dan Phillips PhD

~DEDICATION~

~LARRY~

For your unwavering support, encouragement, and friendship. Your presence in my life has been a constant source of inspiration. Thank you for your invaluable kindness and belief in my journey. This book is a token of appreciation for your enduring friendship and steadfast encouragement.

TABLE OF CONTENT

CREATES AN OPTIMAL ENVIRONMENT FOR HAIR REGROWTH

PART VIII: DIY AYURVEDIC HAIR CARE RECIPES

8. DIY AYURVEDIC HAIR CARE RECIPES

PRACTICAL, STEP-BY-STEP INSTRUCTIONS FOR CREATING HOMEMADE HAIR CARE TREATMENTS USING THE SEVEN AYURVEDIC HERBS

HAIR MASKS, OILS, AND RINSES THAT READERS CAN EASILY PREPARE AND INCORPORATE INTO THEIR HAIR CARE ROUTINES

CHAPTER 1

Introduction to Ayurvedic Hair Care

In a world where contemporary hair care products abound and promise instant cures and amazing changes, the ancient knowledge of Ayurveda provides a welcome diversion. The ancient Indian system of natural medicine known as Ayurveda lays a strong focus on balance and total well-being. This chapter explores the historical significance of Ayurvedic herbs in promoting healthy, vibrant hair as well as the origins of this holistic approach to hair care.

The Core of Ayurveda: Harmony in All Aspects

At the heart of Ayurvedic philosophy is the idea of mind-body-spirit balance. In contrast to traditional methods, which frequently focus only on symptoms, Ayurveda views health as a delicate balance that transcends materiality. Ayurvedic concepts divide people into three "doshas" (individual constitutions): Vata, Pitta, and Kapha. Each dosha is a particular combination of elemental energy. The foundation of Ayurvedic medicine is this individualized approach, which directs everything from lifestyle and nutrition decisions to—most importantly—hair care.

Head Care with Ayurveda: Going Beyond the Surface

In Ayurveda, hair is seen as an extension of the body's general well-being rather than anything separate. While hair problems indicate underlying imbalances, a healthy scalp and shiny hair are thought to be signs of a balanced system. Ayurvedic hair care focuses on treating the underlying causes of hair-related problems rather than just masking the symptoms. This viewpoint is in perfect harmony with Ayurveda's all-encompassing method, which seeks to bring life back from the inside out.

Retracing the History of Herbal Medicine

The history of Ayurveda is rich with references to the medicinal use of herbs. Traditional healers have used the abundance of nature for thousands of years to improve health and cure illnesses. This innate knowledge is demonstrated by the historical importance of Ayurvedic herbs in hair care. There are numerous references to herbal treatments for healthy hair in anything from Ayurvedic books to ancient scrolls.

Amla: The Hair Elixir Found in Nature

Sometimes referred to as Indian gooseberry, Amla is one of the most highly valued herbs in Ayurveda. Amla, which is high in antioxidants and vitamin C, is essential to Ayurvedic hair care. It is said to fortify hair strands, feed hair follicles, and delay the onset of graying. Amla has been used historically for millennia; there are stories of its use helping sages and kings keep their glossy hair.

Bhringraj: The Tonic of Tresses

A noteworthy addition to the Ayurvedic herb repertoire is

Bhringraj, also known as the "King of Hair Herbs." The historical value of Bhringraj is closely linked to its capacity to promote scalp blood circulation. Hair follicles are nourished by this increased blood flow, which encourages hair thickness and growth. Bhringraj has long been praised for its ability to prevent premature balding and hair loss.

Aloe Vera: The Calming Effect of Nature

Aloe Vera is a succulent plant with many uses, and its calming embrace extends beyond skincare. Aloe Vera has a long history of use in many cultures to balance oil production, soothe irritated scalps, and promote healthy conditions for hair development. Its cooling qualities provide relief for irritated scalps, demonstrating Ayurveda's dedication to overall health.

The Path Ahead: Holistically Cultivating Hair

Whereas people are always looking for quick fixes and instant results, Ayurvedic hair care offers a different kind of approach. It encourages people to become back in tune with their own bodies and the rhythms of the natural world. The historical importance of Ayurvedic herbs in supporting hair health serves as a reminder that the knowledge from the past is still applicable now. We are reminded as we set out on this exploration of Ayurvedic hair care that harmony between the mind, body, and spirit is the foundation for both beauty and well-being.

The seven essential Ayurvedic herbs that have withstood the test of time will be examined in the ensuing chapters, along with their amazing qualities and the keys to producing vibrant, healthy hair. The historical significance of each herb and its function in encouraging hair growth will act as a link between traditional knowledge and modern goals for vibrant, radiant hair.

CHAPTER 2

Understanding Hair Loss and Scalp Conditions: Explore the various causes of hair loss, including baldness, alopecia, and thinning. Explain how factors like genetics, lifestyle, and environmental influences contribute to these conditions.

Hair is more than just a physical characteristic; it frequently has deep cultural and symbolic meaning and can represent identity, beauty, and even personality. But the start of hair loss and scalp issues is a disturbing reality for many people. In Chapter 2, the complex world of hair loss is explored, with an emphasis on its causes, symptoms, and contributing factors. The goal of this chapter is to give readers a thorough grasp of the complex relationship between heredity, lifestyle, and environmental factors and how they interact to cause hair loss and scalp disorders.

The Wide Range of Complexity in Hair Loss

The phenomenon of hair loss is complex and includes a range of disorders with different underlying causes and symptoms. While some people naturally lose some hair each day as a result of the hair growth cycle, excessive and obvious hair loss may be a sign of a more serious issue. This chapter examines and clarifies the contributing elements to the emergence of some of the most prevalent types of hair loss, such as baldness, alopecia, and thinning.

Genetics: The Hair Health Blueprint

Genetics is one of the main factors influencing hair health and loss. Studies have demonstrated that an individual's genetic composition accounts for a considerable amount of their susceptibility to different types of hair loss. By affecting variables including hair follicle size, density, and hormone sensitivity, the inheritance of specific genes can raise the risk of hair loss. For example, genetic factors have a major role in the development of androgenetic alopecia, sometimes referred to as male and female pattern baldness. This type of hair loss has a characteristic pattern, with certain areas of the scalp more likely to experience hair thinning and receding hairlines.

Lifestyle Decisions: The Significance of Daily Routines

Apart from heredity, lifestyle decisions have a significant impact on the health and amount of hair lost. Conditions affecting the scalp and hair loss have been related to poor diet, stress, smoking, and heavy alcohol use. In order to support healthy hair growth, the chapter stresses the significance of a balanced diet full of vital vitamins, minerals, and proteins. Chronic stress can also interfere with the normal cycle of hair development, resulting in disorders such as telogen effluvium, in which a significant proportion of hair follicles prematurely reach the resting phase and then shed.

Environmental Impacts: Handling Outside Influences

An individual's living environment has a big influence on their hair health. Exposure to chemicals, pollutants, and UV radiation can cause damage and loss of hair. Hair loss can also be made worse by some jobs that expose workers to harsh chemicals or bad weather all the time. The chapter explores the significance of taking preventative actions, such as utilizing hair products that act as a barrier against environmental stresses and styling hair in a way that reduces exposure to harmful substances.

Differential Hormonal Effects: Hair-Body Association

Hormones are powerful messengers in the body that have a significant impact on hair health. Hair loss can be brought on by changes in hormone levels, such as those that happen during pregnancy, childbirth, menopause, and thyroid conditions. Because of their effect on hair follicles, androgenic hormones, such as testosterone and its derivative dihydrotestosterone

(DHT), are especially linked to hair loss. The chapter delves into the intricate relationship between hair development and hormonal fluctuations, emphasizing the need to consult a physician if you suspect any underlying hormonal problems.

Medical Disorders and Therapy: Handling Contributing Factors

Hair loss and scalp issues can be caused by a variety of medical conditions. The immune system attacks hair follicles in autoimmune illnesses such alopecia areata, resulting in abrupt hair loss in specific places. Chemotherapy and other medical therapies for cancer frequently cause temporary hair loss because they affect rapidly dividing cells, including hair follicles. The need of comprehending these underlying causes and obtaining expert advice to treat hair loss in the context of more general health issues is emphasized throughout the chapter.

Result: A Comprehensive Strategy for Hair Health

To sum up, Chapter 2 clarifies the complex network of variables that lead to scalp disorders and hair loss. A person's genetics determines their susceptibility to different types of hair loss, but environmental factors, medical issues, hormone fluctuations, and lifestyle decisions all affect how well their hair grows. Understanding this complex interaction allows people to take a holistic approach to hair care that includes healthy eating, managing stress, taking precautions against environmental stressors, and seeking medical attention when needed.

In the end, the chapter emphasizes the significance of having a comprehensive understanding of scalp disorders and hair loss, going beyond cosmetic issues to address the underlying reasons. With the right information, people can take charge of their hair health, accept who they are, and face the difficulties of hair loss head-on with courage and self-assurance.

CHAPTER 3

Ayurvedic Principles for Hair Regrowth: Dive into the core principles of Ayurveda that guide its approach to hair care. Explain the concept of doshas (Vata, Pitta, Kapha) and how imbalances can affect hair health.

The pursuit of radiant hair in Ayurvedic medicine goes beyond superficial beauty and into the depths of overall well-being. This chapter explores the deep principles of Ayurvedic hair care, providing an understanding of the doshas (Vata, Pitta, and Kapha) and their dynamic interaction with regard to hair health. As we work through the complex web of Ayurvedic principles, we start to see how imbalances in these elemental energies might impact our hair's health.

Achieving Equilibrium: The Trishas

The idea of doshas, or elemental energies that control our mental, emotional, and physical characteristics, is central to Ayurveda. Vata is a symbol for mobility and change and is connected to air and ether. Pitta, representing both fire and water, is associated with metamorphosis and metabolism. As an indication of solidity and structure, kapha is based in earth and water. Every person has a different blend of these doshas that together comprise their Prakriti, or constitution.

Doshas and Hair Health: The Complex Dance

In the same way that the doshas influence our personalities and physical characteristics, they are also very important for the health of our hair. According to Ayurveda, the body's proper functioning, including that of the hair follicles, depends on the doshas being in a harmonious balance. Any imbalance in the doshas can cause the hair's natural development cycle to be disturbed, which can result in a number of problems like premature greying, thinning, or hair loss.

Hair that is brittle and dry due to vata imbalance

Vata dosha is associated with characteristics of dryness, coolness, and movement. A surplus of Vata might show up as dry, brittle hair that is easily broken. Healthy hair development may be further impeded by a dry and flaky scalp. Ayurveda suggests nourishing and moisturizing therapies that give hair and scalp the essential hydration and stability to counteract Vata imbalance.

Imbalance of Pitta: Overheating and Inflammation

The fiery and transforming Pitta dosha can cause the body to overheat and become inflamed. An unbalanced Pitta can lead to an inflammatory and irritated scalp, which may weaken the hair follicles. Pitta excess is also linked to premature greying and hair thinning. In order to balance Pitta and restore the natural equilibrium of the scalp and hair, it is recommended to apply cooling and calming therapies.

Kapha Imbalance: Weight and Congestion

Qualities of wetness, stability, and heaviness are associated with the kapha dosha. An imbalance in Kapha can cause the scalp to become too oily and congested, which may obstruct hair follicles. This may impede the development of new hair and exacerbate hair loss. Ayurveda recommends cleansing, circulation-boosting, and oil-reducing therapies to alleviate Kapha overload.

Radializing Doses to Promote Hair Growth

The goal of Ayurveda is to bring the body's systems into balance and harmony. The doshas also need to be in balance for the healthiest hair possible. Knowing one's Prakriti, or individual doshic constitution, and correcting any imbalances are essential to encouraging hair growth and keeping vibrant locks.

Personalized Ayurvedic Hair Care: A Customized Method

The customized nature of Ayurvedic hair care concepts is one of its most impressive features. Since every person is different, Ayurveda customizes advice based on a person's doshic constitution and present imbalances. This method explores one's true essence and goes beyond general hair care recommendations.

Wellness for the Whole Person: Hair and Beyond

As we explore the complex terrain of Ayurvedic principles, it becomes clear that general health and hair health are related. The body, mind, and spirit's interior conditions are reflected in the doshas, which act as a mirror. Seeking balance between these elemental elements, we open the door to more vigor, emotional harmony, and mental clarity in addition to shiny hair.

Equipped with knowledge about doshas and their impact on hair health, we set out to investigate seven Ayurvedic plants known for their restorative qualities in the upcoming chapters. We discover a holistic method of hair treatment that not only revitalizes the hair but also feeds the whole being by balancing these herbs with the doshas.

CHAPTER 4

The Power of Ayurvedic Herbs: Introduce the seven key Ayurvedic herbs renowned for promoting hair regrowth. Provide detailed information about each herb's properties, benefits, and historical usage in traditional medicine.

Within the realm of alternative medicine, Ayurveda is a revered, all-encompassing method of healing that dates back many centuries. In Chapter 4, the world of Ayurvedic herbs is explored, and seven important botanical jewels that have gained recognition for their extraordinary capacity to stimulate hair regeneration are revealed. These herbs, which have their roots in ancient wisdom, provide a harmonic and natural way to treat hair loss and grow back luscious, colorful hair. The effectiveness of Ayurvedic knowledge in promoting healthy hair is demonstrated in this chapter by examining the special qualities, advantages, and historical significance of each herb.

First, Bhringraj (Eclipta alba): The Hair Rejuvenation Elixir

Bhringraj, known as the "king of herbs" for hair, has strong hair-rejuvenating effects and is highly regarded in Ayurveda. Bhringraj, which is abundant in vital nutrients and chemicals including wedelolactone and ecliptine, strengthens hair follicles, improves blood flow to the scalp, and delays the onset of gray hair. It has been used historically to treat scalp problems, balding, and hair loss. Made from its leaves, bhringraj oil is a well-liked treatment for massaging the scalp to promote hair growth.

Amla (Emblica officinalis): The Nutritious Scalp Supplement

The Indian gooseberry, or amla, is a plethora of antioxidants, vitamins, and minerals that support healthy hair growth and nourish the scalp. Because of its high vitamin C content, it helps to produce collagen, which strengthens hair and keeps it from breaking. Amla also lessens dandruff and guards against fungal infections by preserving the pH balance of the scalp. Amla is a traditional hair conditioner and luster enhancer that also promotes healthy hair development and leaves hair with a brilliant sheen.

3. Brahmi (Bacopa monnieri): The Hair Rejuvenator for the Mind-Body

Brahmi, well known for its ability to improve cognitive function, is also a potent hair care remedy. This herb lessens worry and stress, two things that are known to cause hair loss. Healthy hair development is indirectly supported by Brahmi, which also balances hormones and calms the mind. Moreover, the phytochemicals in brahmi strengthen hair follicles, lessen hair thinning, and improve circulation on the scalp. With its all-encompassing approach to health, Brahmi creates an atmosphere that's ideal for healthy hair growth.

4. The Guardian Angel of the Scalp: Neem (Azadirachta indica)

Renowned for its antimicrobial and antifungal qualities, neem is a great protector for the scalp. Because of its capacity to fight off scalp infections and lessen inflammation, it fosters the ideal environment for hair follicle growth. Ayurvedic treatments frequently employ neem oil, which is made from the seeds of the neem tree, to cleanse the scalp and encourage hair growth. Neem's effectiveness in preserving a healthy scalp ecology is attested to by its long history of usage in Ayurvedic medicine.

5. Reetha (Sapindus mukorossi): The Miracle of Gentle Cleaning

Reetha, also referred to as soapnut, is a mild yet efficient hair and scalp cleanser. Reetha, being high in saponins, creates a pure lather that removes impurities without depleting the scalp of its natural oils. Properly balanced and clean scalps encourage unrestricted hair development. The use of reetha in Ayurvedic hair care products now is consistent with its historical use as a natural hair cleaner and conditioner.

6. Acacia concinna, or Shikakai: The Secret to Softening Hair

For ages, people have treasured shikakai, sometimes known as "fruit for hair," due to its ability to thicken and smooth hair. Rich in antioxidants and vitamins A, C, and D, shikakai nourishes hair follicles to encourage hair growth and decrease hair loss. In addition, it helps keep the environment around the scalp healthy, preventing dandruff and irritation. Because of its mild nature, shikakai is a recommended option for anyone looking for natural hair washing and conditioning products.

7. Withania somnifera, or ashwagandha: The Stress-Relieving Herbal for Hair Resilience

Renowned adaptogenic herb ashwagandha is essential for stress reduction and general wellbeing. Its effects on stress relief and cortisol reduction are directly related to the health of your hair. It is well known that long-term stress can throw off the cycle of hair growth and cause hair loss. Through the promotion of a well-balanced stress response, ashwagandha indirectly supports the growth of healthy hair. Its importance as a comprehensive hair care solution is highlighted by its historical use in Ayurvedic medicine.

Chapter 4 concludes by praising the deep knowledge of Ayurvedic herbs in encouraging hair growth. By addressing different facets of hair health, these seven botanical treasures—Bhringraj, Amla, Brahmi, Neem, Reetha, Shikakai, and Ashwagandha—offer a comprehensive strategy for fostering healthy hair. Originating from age-old customs and supported by contemporary studies, these herbs represent the harmonious combination of nature and science, offering an all-natural, efficacious, and long-lasting route to lustrous, vivid hair.

CHAPTER 5

Amla: The Nourishing Elixir for Hair: Devote a chapter to Amla (Indian Gooseberry) and its exceptional hair-enhancing properties. Discuss how Amla can strengthen hair follicles, prevent premature greying, and improve overall hair texture.

Amla, sometimes referred to as Indian Gooseberry, is a precious gem among Ayurvedic herbs, valued for its remarkable ability to nourish and remodel hair. This chapter explores the amazing qualities of Amla, including how it can strengthen hair follicles, prevent premature greying, and give hair texture a new lease on life.

The Legacy of Amla: An Age-Old Cure for Contemporary Hair Problems

Amla has been considered sacred in the history of Ayurvedic hair treatment for ages. Its historical significance is entwined with tradition, since it has long been seen as a symbol of longevity and health. Hailed as a hair-enhancing elixir by both sages and kings, Amla's reputation has endured the test of time and grown to become an essential part of modern hair care regimens.

Formulating Hair Follicles: Increasing Inner Strength

The power of amla is found in its large store of nutrients. Amla revitalizes the hair follicles from the inside out by infusing them with nutrients and being rich in vitamin C, antioxidants, and critical minerals. This nutrition prevents hair thinning and breakage by strengthening the follicles and promoting hair growth.

Fighting Early Greying: Amla's Powerful Antioxidant Armour

The onset of early greying can be depressing, but Amla provides a strong protection against this inevitable process. Amla's antioxidants combat free radicals, which are a major cause of premature aging and hair graying. You may give your locks a defense against oxidative stresses that might prematurely fade their color by adding Amla into your hair care regimen.

Beautiful Texture: Increasing the Aesthetic Appeal of Hair

The advantages of amla go beyond its ability to nourish and protect. It has the special power to improve the texture of hair, leaving it silkier, smoother, and easier to manage. Through the treatment of frizz, roughness, and dullness, Amla makes hair shine like a brilliant crown of beauty.

Amala in Operation: Submission and Integration

It is possible to use Amla's potential for hair care in a number of ways. Extracted from the fruit's extract, amla oil is a well-liked option for deep conditioning and massage. By rubbing Amla oil into the scalp, you can increase blood flow, which helps the hair follicles receive vital nutrients. Amla-derived hair masks, powders, and rinses provide flexible options that let people customize their use according to their specific hair needs.

The Path to Shining Hair: Consistency and Patience

To fully benefit from Amla's benefits for hair health, like with any natural cure, patience and persistence are required. Even though the benefits of amla might not show up right once, they are based on overall wellbeing. By include amla in your hair care routine, you're taking a journey that reflects the ideals of Ayurveda: nourishing from the inside out, balancing the body and mind, and accepting the knowledge of the natural world.

Amla's Call: A Comprehensive Metamorphosis

We accept an invitation to a comprehensive metamorphosis that goes beyond hair health when we embrace Amla's nourishing elixir. We reestablish contact with traditional knowledge that recognizes the unity of the body, mind, and spirit. Amla's nutrients give each strand of hair life while its antioxidants fortify the durability of our hair. And we recognize the beauty that arises when we accept nature's gifts with appreciation and purpose as we run our fingers through our restored hair.

The story of Ayurvedic hair care is further revealed in the ensuing chapters, which all focus on the special qualities of botanical marvels that have been used for generations to revitalize hair. We set out on a voyage through nature's garden of hair-enhancing treasures, from Bhringraj to Aloe Vera, discovering the secrets they offer for people looking for vibrant, robust, and genuinely gorgeous hair.

CHAPTER 6

Bhringraj: The King of Hair Herbs: Explore the significance of Bhringraj in Ayurveda and its role in treating hair loss and promoting regrowth. Highlight its effectiveness in improving blood circulation to the scalp and stimulating hair follicles.

Within the field of Ayurveda, an age-old holistic medical approach that prioritizes equilibrium and health, Bhringraj (Eclipta alba) is regarded as the "King of Hair Herbs." Since ancient times, Bhringraj, with its rich historical background and powerful medicinal qualities, has been valued for its exceptional ability to treat hair loss, stimulate regrowth, and maintain general hair health. This chapter explores the importance of Bhringraj in Ayurveda, emphasizing how it can stimulate hair follicles and improve blood circulation to the scalp to revitalize the locks that decorate the human form.

The Historical and Cultural Significance of Bhringraj:

Because of its many advantages, Bhringraj, which means "King of Tresses" in Sanskrit, has been an essential component of Ayurvedic practices. This plant, which has its roots in India, is well-known for its wider health and energy benefits in addition to its ability to improve hair. Bhringraj has long been a mainstay in ancient Ayurvedic formulas meant to treat a variety of illnesses, such as skin issues and liver problems. It's a beloved herb in holistic wellness because of its deep-rooted cultural identification as a symbol of energy and rejuvenation.

Moving Towards Regrowth and Addressing Hair Loss:

The secret to Bhringraj's popularity is its remarkable capacity to treat hair loss and encourage regrowth. Whether brought on by environmental, lifestyle, or hereditary factors, hair loss can cause severe psychological and emotional suffering. Targeting both the underlying reasons and the outward signs of hair loss, Bhringraj provides a natural and comprehensive solution to this issue. In order to provide the ideal environment for hair regrowth, it achieves this by improving blood circulation to the scalp and activating hair follicles.

Stimulation of Hair Follicles and Blood Circulation:

Bhringraj's strong vasodilatory qualities are one of its best qualities. Blood vessels widening, or vasodilation, leads to an increase in blood flow. Bhringraj increases vasodilation in the scalp when given topically or consumed, which enhances blood flow to hair follicles. The hair follicles receive vital nutrients and oxygen from the increased blood flow, which supplies the building blocks required for strong, healthy hair growth. Furthermore, enhanced blood circulation guarantees the effective elimination of waste materials, averting scalp congestion that may hinder the creation of new hair.

Activation of Follicles in the Hair:

Beyond just increasing blood flow, Bhringraj also stimulates hair follicles directly, rousing them from their dormant state. Telogen, or resting phase, is a stage in which hair follicles can experience hair shedding and reduced regrowth. The active ingredients in bhringraj, such as wedelolactone and ecliptine, encourage hair follicles to move from the telogen to the anagen phase, or growth phase. This stimulation efficiently prevents hair thinning and promotes thicker, denser hair by stimulating the growth of new hair strands.

Feeding and Strengthening:

Bhringraj is also a great source of vital nutrients that support the health of hair. Its vitamin, mineral, and antioxidant content strengthens hair shafts, nourishes hair follicles, and improves hair condition overall. By preventing breakage, broken ends, and brittleness, these nutrients promote strong, glossy hair. Bhringraj's all-encompassing method of hair care guarantees that it not only treats hair loss and encourages regrowth but also enhances the tactile and visual qualities of well-maintained hair.

Recap: Bhringraj's Domination in Hairdressing

In conclusion, considering its historical importance and powerful medicinal qualities, Bhringraj is a well-deserved title for the "King of Hair Herbs" in Ayurveda. Its ability to treat hair loss and encourage regrowth is evidence of Ayurveda's holistic teachings, which place an emphasis on the interdependence of all body systems. Bhringraj facilitates healthy hair development by enhancing blood circulation to the scalp and invigorating hair follicles. Bhringraj is the embodiment of Ayurvedic wisdom; it can be taken as oils, powders, or capsules, and it offers a natural and harmonious way to nurture and restore the crowning splendor, which is an essential component of a person's identity and well-being.

CHAPTER 7

Aloe Vera: Soothing Scalp Remedy: Focus on Aloe Vera's soothing and moisturizing effects on the scalp. Discuss how it can alleviate scalp conditions, reduce inflammation, and create an optimal environment for hair regrowth.

Few products in the natural hair care line can compare to Aloe Vera's soft embrace and multifaceted advantages. This chapter explores the calming properties of aloe vera and how it can serve as a haven for the scalp. Aloe Vera is a symbol of nature's curative power because of its multifaceted therapeutic properties, which include reducing inflammation and treating scalp disorders, as well as creating the ideal environment for hair growth.

The Age-Old Legacy of Aloe Vera: An Everlasting Calming Agent

The long history of aloe vera as a calming plant transcends centuries and cultures. Its historical significance is second only to that of gel; records of its use stretch back thousands of years. The capacity of aloe vera to soothe, calm, and rejuvenate has long been valued, from the sun-kissed plains of Egypt to the verdant vistas of ancient India.

Scalp Chaos Calming: Reducing Scalp Conditions

The scalp, which is frequently disregarded, is the source of healthy hair growth. Aloe Vera is a fantastic treatment for a variety of scalp disorders because of its calming and hydrating qualities. Whether your scalp is dry, itchy, or prone to dandruff, Aloe Vera's moisturizing properties help rebalance and soothe irritated scalps.

The Cooling Effect of Aloe Vera: The Nemesis of Inflammation

Many scalp issues are rooted in inflammation. It can be brought on by environmental stressors, sensitivity, or the aftermath of styling, but Aloe Vera's anti-inflammatory qualities provide a soothing and cool solution. Because of its natural ingredients, it helps to create an environment that promotes healthy scalp function and hair development by reducing redness, swelling, and irritation.

The Oasis for Growth: Promoting Hair Regrowth

The effects of aloe vera go beyond just comfort; it creates an atmosphere that encourages hair development. Because of its enzymatic makeup, which removes dead skin cells and lets air into hair follicles, it gently exfoliates the scalp. By keeping the scalp healthy and balanced, aloe vera promotes the growth of new hair and turns the scalp into a lush haven for hair restoration.

Use and Integration: Aloe Vera Ceremonies

Aloe Vera's adaptability makes it possible to incorporate it easily into a variety of hair care routines. A strong and straightforward remedy is provided by fresh aloe vera gel that is taken straight from the plant. Applying it as a mask or treatment on the scalp enables its revitalizing qualities to deeply penetrate. Commercial aloe vera products provide easy ways to take use of its benefits as well. Examples include shampoos, conditioners, and hair masks.

Embracing the Touch of Nature: A Comprehensive Approach

We discover that Aloe Vera embodies the concept of comprehensive well-being as we delve deeper into its world of calming scalp cures. In the same way that Aloe Vera benefits the scalp, Ayurveda advises us to take care of our body, mind, and soul. Aloe Vera takes on symbolic meaning as a representation of the close relationship between nature and human health, serving as a constant reminder that using natural medicines involves more than just attaining aesthetic beauty—it also entails developing a harmonious relationship with the environment.

The Whisper of Aloe Vera: A Transformational Promise

The whisper of aloe vera holds the possibility of metamorphosis—a trip from agitation to release, from discomfort to serenity, and from stagnation to regeneration. We access ancient knowledge that is in harmony with the cycles of the natural world when we use Aloe Vera into our hair care regimens. We rejoice in the earth's healing power as it performs wonders on our scalp, hair, and general wellbeing with every application.

As we continue our investigation into nature's remedy for healthy hair, we follow Aloe Vera as our guide. We move from the comforting embrace of aloe vera to the thrilling discoveries that lie ahead in the world of botanical marvels. Every chapter reveals the secrets of plants that have traveled through time, sharing their abundance with those who want hair that is vibrant, strong, and genuinely amazing.

CHAPTER 8

DIY Ayurvedic Hair Care Recipes: Provide readers with practical, step-by-step instructions for creating homemade hair care treatments using the seven Ayurvedic herbs. Include hair masks, oils, and rinses that readers can easily prepare and incorporate into their hair care routines.

With the help of these seven essential Ayurvedic herbs, you can discover the age-old secrets of Ayurvedic hair care. You may incorporate natural ingredients into your hair care routine by making DIY hair masks, oils, and rinses with the help of these helpful and simple-to-follow guidelines. Bid adieu to chemical-laden commercial hair products and hello to Ayurvedic holistic wisdom.

1. Hair Oil of Bhringraj:

Ingredients: - 1/2 cup fresh or dried Bhringraj leaves - 1 cup coconut oil

1. To liberate the natural oils from the Bhringraj leaves, crush them.

2. Put the coconut oil and crushed leaves in a heat-resistant basin.

3. Use a double boiler or microwave to warm the mixture until the Bhringraj essence is fully absorbed into the oil. Allow to cool.

4. To ensure no leaf residue remains, strain the oil.

5. Gently massage the oil into your hair and scalp. Keep it on for the entire night or for at least an hour.

6. Use a light Ayurvedic shampoo to wash and rinse.

2. Hair Mask with Shikakai and Amla:

Components: - Two tablespoons of Amla powder

2-tablespoons of shikakai powder

Amount of yogurt required to create a paste

Guidelines:

In a bowl, combine the powders of Amla and Shikakai.

2. Gradually add yogurt to make a paste that is smooth.

3. Focus on the scalp and individual hair strands when applying the mask to moist hair.

Let it run for thirty to forty-five minutes.

5. Give your hair a good rinse and shampoo.

3. Scalp Rinse with Brahmi and Neem:

Components:

– 2 tablespoons Brahmi powder

- Two tablespoons of neem powder

- Aqua

Directions: 1. In a bowl, combine the powders of brahmi and neem.

2. Include enough water to make a paste that is thin.

3. Create portions in your hair and massage the paste into your scalp.

4. After a light massage, leave it for ten to fifteen minutes.

5. Give your scalp a good rinse, then use a light shampoo.

4. Shampoo for Hair by Reetha:

Components:

Soapnut (Reetha) shells, five to six

Two cups of water

1. Use a mallet to break up the Reetha shells into smaller pieces.

2. Bring the crushed Reetha shells to a boil in water for approximately 20 minutes, or until a soapy solution forms.

3. After the solution has cooled, strain it to get rid of any remaining shell.

4. Cleanse your hair naturally with the Reetha solution. After giving your scalp and hair a gentle massage, completely rinse.

5. Stress-Relieving Hair Mask with Ashwagandha:

Contains: - Two tablespoons of ashwagandha powder

(As needed to form a paste) - Coconut milk

Guidelines:

1. To make a paste, combine coconut milk and ashwagandha powder.

2. Dab the paste into your hair and scalp.

3. Shut it off after 30 to 45 minutes.

4. Give your hair a good rinse and shampoo.

6. Hair Growth Oil with Bhringraj and Amla:

Ingredients: - 1/4 cup handmade or premade Bhringraj oil

1 tablespoon powdered amla

Guidelines:

1. In a bowl, combine the amla powder and Bhringraj oil.

2. Use a microwave or double boiler to gently reheat the mixture.

3. After letting it cool, strain it to get rid of any particles.

4. Work the oil mixture into your hair and scalp. For a few hours or overnight, leave it on.

5. Use a light Ayurvedic shampoo to wash and rinse.

7. Aloe Vera and Brahmi Hair Conditioning Mask:

Components: - Two tablespoons of Brahmi powder
(As needed to produce a paste) - Aloe vera gel

Guidelines:

1. To make a paste, combine aloe vera gel and brahmi powder.

2. Apply the paste to your hair, paying special attention to the ends and lengths.

3. Shut it off after 30 to 45 minutes.

4. Give your hair a good rinse and shampoo.

You may maximize the health, strength, and vitality of your hair by implementing these seven essential herbs into your routine for DIY Ayurvedic hair care. Try out these natural remedies to see which ones work best for you, and accept the holistic approach to hair care that Ayurveda has to offer.